Heal Your Headache

The Ultimate Guide to Eliminating and Reducing your Headache Naturally!

Heal your Headache

Healthy Body Books

http://www.healthybodybooks.com

ISBN-13:
978-1501038396

ISBN-10:
1501038397

This document is geared towards providing exact and
reliable information in regards to the topic and issue
covered. The publication is sold with the idea that the
publisher is not required to render accounting, officially
permitted, or otherwise, qualified services. If advice is
necessary, legal or professional, a practiced individual in
the profession should be ordered.

The author of this book does not dispense medical
advice or prescribe the use of any technique as a form of

treatment for physical, emotional, or medical problems without the advice of a physician, either directly or indirectly. The intent of the author is only to offer information of a general nature to help you in your quest for emotional, spiritual and physical well-being. In the event you use any of the information in this book for yourself, which is your constitutional right, the author and the publisher assume no responsibility for your actions. Under no circumstances will any legal responsibility or blame be held against the publisher for any reparation, damages, or monetary loss due to the information herein, either directly or indirectly.

The information herein is offered for informational purposes solely, and is universal as so. The presentation of the information is without contract or any type of guarantee assurance.

The trademarks that are used are without any consent, and the publication of the trademark is without permission or backing by the trademark owner. All trademarks and brands within this book are for clarifying purposes only and are the owned by the owners themselves, not affiliated with this document.

Table Of Contents

Introduction

Are you worried you'll never be free from Headaches?

Are you sick of pesky headaches ruling your life?

Have you had such a bad headaches you've been stuck in bed for days?

Have you missed a special Occasion just because of a Headache?

Do you just wish you knew how to manage or eliminate your Headaches?

In this book you will discover the most up-to-date information on healing Headaches including:

-What is a Headache

-What types of headaches are there?

-Natural treatments for headaches

-Reducing the Pain

And much more!

I want to thank you and congratulate you for buying this book, "Heal Your Headache: The Ultimate Guide to Reducing and Eliminating your Headache Naturally!"

Taking the first step is sometimes half of the battle!

My name is Simone, and I am the creator of the Healthy Body Books. I would like to take this opportunity to tell you who I am and why I decided to create this helpful tool.

My passion for health extends beyond the superficial. A part of me has always been called to make health a priority in my life. I am dedicated to making my body perfect, at least the way I see it.

Unfortunately, one change in my routine made it that much harder to obtain the perfect body. I found myself not feeling as good as I used to, and I even felt like I could not longer achieve my goals. To put it bluntly, I was concerned for my health and my future.

After searching long and hard for potential solutions to my problem, I found relief in changing my diet, natural therapies and self-help. Using a number of natural techniques, I was finally able to get my life back under control – and it felt great! I felt like things were really the way they were supposed to be.

If you are trying to find another way to stay healthy, the Healthy Body Books are meant for you. If you feel like something in your life just isn't working and might even be stopping you from living the life you want to live, you will find solace in new techniques and knowledge. Each book is written by experts, but the everyday person will be able to read and the books with ease.

Good luck!

Keep Up to Date with New Releases

Thank you again for grabbing yourself a copy of this Book Heal Your Headache: The Ultimate Guide to Reducing and Eliminating your Headache Naturally!

I'd like to reward you with this by offering you access to my others books for free by joining my newsletter!

You will be getting up to date information on health, fitness and diet, and also get access to getting other Healthy Body Books for free. By joining my newsletter you will be taking a big step forward in being your Healthiest Body yet!

Just visit **http://www.healthybodybooks.com** and get free instant access to the Healthy Body Books newsletter today!

Lastly once you finish reading this book would please review this book on Amazon. With your feedback I continue to make this book better and better.

Thank you.

Chapter 1: What is Headache?

Headache is a very common disorder that almost every one may experience at one point in life. It is characterized by varying levels of pain on a part or parts of the head.

When you feel a mild headache, you may tend to immediately take over-the-counter medicines. These over-the-counter medicines usually take away the pain in just a few minutes to an hour.

When the headache becomes worse or unbearable, it may cause the you to have some difficulty or totally prevent you from doing your usual tasks. It may even cause you to miss work or school.

Headaches can be categorized into two groups: primary and secondary headaches.

Primary headaches are those which are not caused by any other illness.

Secondary headaches are those which are caused by another health condition.

Secondary headaches can be caused by a concussion, a head injury, drinking alcohol, flu, a cold, sinusitis or allergic reaction.

There are also several types of headache: tension headache, migraine, sinus headache, cluster headache, medication headache, temporomandibular joint disorders, hormone headache or giant cell arteritis.

A mild headache can usually be relieved by just taking more fluids or getting enough rest.

Over-the-counter pain relievers can heal your mild to moderate headaches.

If a head pain persists or is getting worse, it could be a sign of an underlying illness or a more serious disorder. If this happens, it is best that you seek the medical advice of a trusted doctor or health care professional.

When a headache occurs suddenly and severely, it could also be a sign of another illness. You must consult a doctor for medical attention and diagnosis.

It is also best to get medical assistance immediately if you get the headache after a blow to your head or an accident.

A headache which is accompanied by pain in the ear or eye, stiff neck, loss of consciousness, fever and confusion might also be a sign of a more serious illness. It is best to seek the help of a doctor immediately.

Chapter 2: Types of Headache: Tension Headache

Headache is categorized into different types. One of these is the tension type headache.

Tension headache is usually experienced by most people at one point in their life.

A tension headache is characterized by a mild ache and pressure on the top, front and sides of the head.

Causes of Tension Headache

Tension headache can be caused by the tightening of the muscles in either the neck, shoulders, jaw or scalp.

It can also be caused by emotional or mental problems such as anxicty, stress or depression.

Overworking can also cause tension headache.

Lack of rest or inadequate amount of sleep can also cause this type of headache.

Hunger or missing a meal can also cause a tension-type headache.

Dehydration can also be a cause of a tension headache.

A hangover after drinking alcohol can also be another cause.

Poor posture can also cause tension headache because it strains the muscles of the shoulders.

Noise and bright lighting can also cause tension headache, as well as strong or offensive odors.

Lack of exercise can also be a possible cause. It is due to the poor blood circulation and strained muscles which might then cause a tension headache.

Who Are Affected By Tension Headache?

Most people can experience this type of headache.

It is more common in adults and adolescents, but it can also happen at any age.

Women also tend to have greater chances of getting tension headaches than men based on some studies.

Warning Signs of Tension Headache

A tension headache does not usually need medical attention but if it happens more often, it is best to consult a doctor.

Some other warning signs that may tell you to immediately seek medical advice when:

Your headache is accompanied by fever, stiff neck, confusion and vomiting;

It is much different than your previous headaches and is sudden;

You feel numbness, weakness, confusion and speech difficulty;

11

It comes after a blow to the head or an accident.

You must immediately seek the doctor's advice because these symptoms may indicate a more serious condition.

Treatment for Tension Headache

Tension headaches are usually not that serious and can be treated by taking painkillers such as ibuprofen, aspirin and paracetamol.

The use of painkillers must be used with caution in pregnant women and in children below 16 because these can cause some future health problems.

Some natural treatments can also cure this type of headache.

Massaging, yoga, relaxation and hot compress are common natural cures for headache caused by stress.

Exercising regularly and practicing a good posture can also be a good way to avoid tension headaches.

Proper hydration and getting adequate rest are also key to avoid headaches.

Some people use acupuncture techniques to cure chronic tension headaches.

Amitriptyline, an anti-depressant, can also be used in some cases of chronic tension headaches.

Chapter 3: Types of Headache: Migraine

Migraine is a less common type of headache.

Migraine attacks can come frequently or occasionally.

Symptoms of Migraine

The head pain caused by migraine can be characterized by recurrent headache and it may even prevent you from doing your normal day-to-day activities.

Migraine can also be characterized by a throbbing or pounding pain on either or both sides of your head.

Some of the other symptoms of migraine include sensitivity to lights and nausea.

Migraine can interfere with the daily activities of one person so treatment is very much needed.

Stages of Migraine

Migraine has five stages. Despite of having migraine, not all people may experience all of these stages.

Prodomal Stage - This is the first stage of migraine. During this stage, you may experience some changes in energy level, vitality, mood, pain, appetite and behavior before a migraine attack arises.

Aura Stage - This is a stage before the migraine attack starts. Symptoms during this stage include some disparities in vision such as difficulty in focusing, blind spots or flashes of light. These symptoms can last for a few minutes to one hour.

Headache Stage - This is the stage of migraine in which you may experience the pain or throbbing sensation on either side of the head. It can be accompanied by vomiting, nausea and oversensitivity to loud sounds and bright lights. These symptoms can last for up to 3 days.

Resolution Stage - It is the stage in which the pain subsides. In some cases, the pain can stop suddenly. While in others, the pain can stop gradually. Relaxing and sleeping can help in relieving the pain.

Recovery or Postdromal Stage - This is the stage in which you may experience weakness and exhaustion.

Types of Migraine

There are also different types of migraine.

Migraine Without Aura - It is the type of migraine in which there is headache but without symptoms of aura.

Migraine Without Headache - This type of migraine is also called *silent migraine*. In this type, you may experience aura and other symptoms of migraine but without the headache.

Migraine With Aura - It is the type of migraine in which you may experience different symptoms and aura before the headache starts. Symptoms may include tightening of shoulder and neck muscles, hypersensitivity to lights and other visual problems.

Who Are Affected By Migraine?

Migraine can affect anyone. But it affects more people under the age of 40.

Causes of Migraine

Migraine can be triggered by certain foods and stress.

It can also be caused by hormonal changes. Some women may experience migraine during their menstrual period.

Treatment for Migraine

There are some over-the-counter medications which can effectively cure the pain caused by migraine.

However, more potent prescription medicines are used for more severe migraine.

Chapter 4: Types of Headache: Cluster Headache

Cluster type is another kind of headache.

Cluster type is also classified as a primary headache.

It is also called a *suicidal headache* because it is characterized by severe head pain.

Symptoms of Cluster Headache

Cluster headaches are characterized by excruciating head pain which can radiate around an eye or behind it.

Pain from cluster headaches is much worse than other types of headache.

Cluster headaches are rare. These can come unexpectedly. These can happen in clusters for a period of a month or two at a certain times of the year.

People who suffer from cluster headaches sometimes rock or bump their heads against a wall because of the uncomfortable and unbearable pain.

Types of Cluster Headache

Cluster headaches can be either episodic or chronic.

Episodic cluster headaches can last for a certain period and stop for more than a month then come back for another period.

Chronic cluster headaches can last for a long time and can stop for less than a month or not at all.

Causes of Cluster Headache

Cluster headaches are believed to be caused by the activity of hypothalamus in the brain. It is caused by the expanding of blood vessels which causes pressure.

It can also be aggravated by alcohol intake during headache attacks.

It can also be triggered by extreme temperature changes.

Inhalation of nitroglycerin, a chemical which is known to expand blood vessels, is also believed to trigger cluster headaches.

Cluster headaches are common during spring and fall.

Treatment for Cluster Headache

Cluster headaches might not be treated with over-the-counter medications. These headaches can only be treated by certain prescription drugs.

Sumatriptan and oxygen therapy are some of the treatments for cluster headaches.

Chapter 5: Types of Headache: Sinus Headaches

An infected sinus is the main cause of sinus headache. Sinus headache is uncommon.

Symptoms of Sinus Headache

Sinus headache is characterized by a faint but throbbing pain on the upper part of the face.

Sinus headache is often mistaken for tension headache or migraine.

A throbbing and constant pain in the face is a sign of sinus headache. It is usually felt on the upper teeth or under the eyes.

The pain from sinus headache is usually worse at the morning. It usually subsides at the afternoon.

Moving the head, bending down or extreme changes from warm to cold temperatures can trigger the sinus pain to become worse.

The face may also be tender to touch and you may also have a runny nose during a sinus headache.

There are some symptoms of a sinus headache which can be similar to a migraine or a tension headache such as sudden or quick movements.

Any severe headache must be consulted with a medical professional to get the proper diagnosis and treatment.

Cause of Sinus Headache

Sinuses are small hollows that are found behind the cheeks, nose and eyes. Sinuses allow the air to circulate normally and the mucus to drain.

When the upper airways and the lining of the nose become swollen and infected, the sinuses can become blocked. When the sinuses are blocked, the mucus cannot be drained and builds up in the sinuses.

Buildup of mucus in the sinuses can cause a feeling of congestion and stuffiness. Once the mucus clears out, these symptoms go away as well.

Another infection can develop when bacteria thrives in the blocked mucus inside the sinuses. This condition is called sinusitis.

When you have sinusitis, too much mucus can build up inside the sinuses. The mucus build up can lead to a painful and intense pressure which is called a sinus headache.

Treatment for Sinus Headache

Sinus headaches are usually treated by taking antihistamines, decongestants or corticosteroids.

Chapter 6: Types of Headache: Hormone Headaches

Changes in the hormone levels of the body may also cause headaches. This usually happens in women. Women may have headaches during their monthly periods, while taking contraceptive pills, during pregnancy or menopause.

Hormone headache is usually experienced by women. Millions of women may experience hormone headache each month according to some research.

Causes of Hormone Headache

Because of the changes in hormone levels during the menstrual period, women are most likely to have hormone headache around this time.

The use of contraceptive pills can also trigger hormone headache. These pills contain hormones that aids in contraception. While some women may not feel headache while taking the pills, they might experience severe headaches during the pill-free week.

The stage of menopause is also another factor that triggers hormone headache. The balance of hormones in the body is disrupted during menopause which may cause severe headaches.

Pregnancy is also a cause of hormone headaches. When a woman gets pregnant, she may experience pregnancy headaches because of the changes in her body and hormones.

These pregnancy headaches may be experienced severely during the first three months of pregnancy. Hormone headache does not affect the baby.

To be able to pinpoint a hormone headache, a person or a woman must keep a note of her headache attacks and menstrual periods. If these headaches usually come during menstruation, it is most likely that it is caused by hormones.

Treatment for Hormone Headache

Eating well, getting enough sleep and avoiding stress can help relieve hormone headache.

If you have a regular period, you can take estrogen supplements to help relieve your headache. It can come in a patch or as a topical gel, which can be prescribed by a doctor.

Migraine medicines such as mefenamic acid or triptan can also help relieve hormone headache.

If your hormone headache is due to the pill-free week (during the use of contraceptive pills), ask your doctor for ways on how to continuously take hormonal contraceptive pills.

If your hormone headache is due to menopause, you can ask your doctor for hormone replacement therapy. It will not only improve your headaches but also treat some of the menopausal symptoms such as flushes. Hormone replacement drugs in the form of patch and gel are better in treating migraines and headaches.

Chapter 7: Types of Headache: Painkiller Headaches

Some medications can cause headaches. Taking too much pain killers can also cause headaches.

Painkillers can cause rebound headaches when used too often. Most of these happen to those who use painkillers as a treatment for headache.

When you take too much of these painkillers, your body becomes immune to the effect. The rebound headache usually shows up when you stop taking the painkillers. It might be because your body has already become dependent to the painkillers.

A rebound headache may also occur when the effect of the painkiller subsides. The cycle will only continue and make the headaches worse.

Causes of Painkiller Headache

Painkillers such as paracetamol, codeine, non-steroidal anti-inflammatory drugs (ibuprofen or aspirin) and anti-migraine drugs or triptans (sumatriptan) can cause this kind of headache.

Treatment for Painkiller Headache

It is important to avoid taking painkillers for two or more consecutive days or more than twice a week.

It is also better to avoid painkillers that contain codeine such as Solpadeine or Syndol.

To effectively stop this kind of headache, you must simply stop taking them. Once you do this, you may experience worse headaches and sickness, but after your system becomes free from the painkiller residue, you will start to feel better.

But do not stop abruptly if you are using codeine and other related drugs, for it may be dangerous. Ask your doctor for advice on how to gradually decrease and stop taking this painkiller.

When you have already cleared out your painkiller headaches, you can use painkillers again for your headaches but only with proper caution.

Chapter 8: Types of Headache: Temporomandibular Joint Disorders

One symptom of TJD or Temporomandibular Joint Disorder is a headache.

The joint between the base of the skull and the lower jaw is affected by TJD.

Although this is not a serious disorder, it can cause difficulty in your daily life.

Who Are Affected By TJD?

About 30% of adults can experience TJD at one point in their life.

Symptoms of TJD

TJD can be accompanied by headache, popping sounds when moving the jaw, pain in the jaw area, ear, temples and cheek, difficulty in opening the mouth and muscle spasms.

Symptoms of TJD can stay for a few months before they disappear.

Causes of TJD

TJD can be caused by teeth grinding, which overuses the muscles and joint of the jaw.

Osteoarthritis, gout or rheumatoid arthritis can also be a cause of TJD.

Jaw or facial injuries can also cause TJD.

Treatment for TJD

For severe cases of TJD, surgery may be needed to treat it.

For less serious cases of TJD, there are some techniques that can be done to treat it:

Jaw stretching exercise followed by a warm compress.

Avoiding chewing gums and eating soft foods only.

Massaging the jaw muscles.

Avoiding to widely open the jaw.

Avoiding to rest the chin on the hand.

Relaxation.

Using mouth guards can also help to stop teeth grinding and clenching.

Pain relievers such as ibuprofen, paracetamol, codeine can also be used. Tricyclic antidepressant or muscle relaxant can be prescribed for more severe cases.

Steroid injections can be more effective for TJDs due to arthritis. The steroid injection can reduce the swelling and pain in the joint. The effect of this treatment can be either temporary or permanent.

Joint replacement can be the best treatment for those with severe cases of TJD. The Temporomandibular joint is replaced by an artificial joint. This surgery is done under general anesthetic. All of the affected joints are replaced.

Arthrocentesis is a process in which a solution is injected into the upper jaw using needles to flush out microparticles and loosen up the joint, is another treatment for TJD.

An open joint surgery may also be done to better inspect the jaw for possible problems or tumors.

Arthroscopy, a surgery in which a cut is made to let an instrument to enter the jaw and allow the doctor to see any abnormality, realign the jaw or remove an inflamed tissue.

Chapter 9: Types of Headache: Giant Cell Arteritis

Giant Cell Arteritis is a disorder in which the large and medium arteries of the neck and head become inflamed. This usually causes headache.

Who Are Affected By Giant Cell Arteritis?

This condition usually affects people at their 60s.

Symptoms of Giant Cell Arteritis

Medical attention is needed in case of Giant Cell Arteritis. Immediate medical help is needed when you:

develop jaw pain while eating

severe headache

sore scalp

double or blurred vision.

Treatment For Giant Cell Arteritis

The use of corticosteroids is the main treatment for giant cell arteritis. This treatment needs to done for two years to prevent the symptoms from recurring.

Immunosuppressant's and low dose aspirins can also be used with corticosteroids to avoid the recurring of symptoms and other complications.

Chapter 10: Natural Ways To Heal Your Headache

People usually take over-the-counter medicines or pain relievers to cure their headache.

Relaxing and taking some time to rest can be an effective way to alleviate a tension headache.

Changing a person's lifestyle can also help in reducing the chances of having headaches.

The following are some natural ways to reduce and eliminate headache:

Cold Flannel - Put a cold flannel on top of your affected sinus or sinuses (in case of a sinus headache) a few times a day. The coolness can help relieve the pain from the pressured sinuses by constricting the blood vessels. When it becomes warm, soak it again in cold water.

For a long lasting cold compress, put a wet towel inside a zip lock bag and pop into the freezer for a few minutes. Take it out and put over the affected area.

Take a Break - Find some place dark and lie down on a bed or couch for a few minutes.

Take a few breaths and relax.

Make sure that you find a quiet place to help you relax and take a short nap.

Adjust the temperature to your preference.

Find a comfortable bed or couch and wear an eye mask to help block out the light.

Rehydrate - Some headaches may be caused by dehydration.

You may get a hangover headache from a drinking session or after you have vomited, you may have lost a lot of fluids and become dehydrated. Drinking a few glasses of water throughout the day can help you to rehydrate, doing this can help ease your headache.

Ginger - Ginger tea can help reduce inflammations, which often cause headaches. Ginger has been well known for a lot of medicinal properties. Simply boil ginger root with water and let it cool. Then drink it as a tea.

Saline Nasal Spray - Although this can be bought at the pharmacy, this over-the-counter medication is milder and more basic compared to other medications. It usually contains salt or sodium chloride dissolved in distilled water.

Douching your nasal canal with this can help lessen the swelling of the sinuses during a sinus headache. It helps in washing out the bacteria, allergens and mucus.

Butterbur - Butterbur extract can also be taken to treat headaches. It can come in forms of tincture, capsule or powder. It has anti-inflammatory and antispasmodic effects.

Take Some Caffeine But Cautiously - Painkillers usually contain caffeine. Caffeine boosts the effect of painkillers and constricts the blood vessels.

But make sure that you drink caffeine with caution. A sudden stop in caffeine consumption can cause you a headache as well.

Also check your painkillers if they already contain caffeine. If so, do not take extra caffeine because it might lead to a rebound headache.

Use A Humidifier - Inhale some moist air from a humidifier, doing this can help clear out and relax the airways during a sinus headache.

Magnesium - Magnesium supplements can be taken to help in calming the nerves. Some people with migraine are diagnosed to have magnesium deficiency. Magnesium can also be found in beans, broccoli, spinach, soy milk and nuts.

Massage - Stimulate circulation by massaging your neck, scalp and earlobes.

Lightly massage them to relieve the tension and pain. gently press your temples and move your finger in slow circles.

You can also massage your scalp while shampooing in the shower or by pouring some argon or coconut oil on your hands and massaging it onto the scalp.

31

You can also apply some pressure on the space between your thumb and index finger for a few minutes on each hand.

You can also ask somebody to massage your back and your neck.

You can also use two tennis balls packed inside a sock. Lie down and put it underneath the base of your skull and relax.

You can also massage your nose bridge to help ease migraine and sinus headaches.

Use hydrotherapy - Hydrotherapy can help improve the blood circulation of the body and release toxins.

Do this by alternately standing in hot and cold water for two minutes each for twenty minutes.

Pray/Meditate - Praying or meditating can help relieve tension by inducing calm and reducing stress and tension. It also helps you to release bad vibes and let go of negative thoughts which triggers your headaches. Find a quiet place, close your eyes and pray.

Visualize - Too much exposure to complicated situations and noises can causes stress and headaches. Try to close your eyes and visualize a peaceful scenery or a happy setting. This can help you calm down, relieve your headache and amp up your mood.

Do Not Strain Your Eyes - Too much staring at the computer monitor can lead to eye strain and headaches. To avoid this, take a few minutes break and stare at something twenty feet away.

You can also adjust the distance and the brightness of the monitor for a much comfortable view.

Apple Cider Vinegar - Apply a compress soaked in vinegar over your aching head.

You can also breathe in some steam with apple cider vinegar.

Mix some of the apple cider vinegar with boiling water in a bowl. Drape a towel over your head to trap the steam. Breath in the steam until the water cools down. Drink some cool water afterwards.

Use Your Sense of Smell - Aromatherapy is a well-known technique to help relieve certain disorders.

Use chamomile, lavender or sweet marjoram oils to treat headaches. You can put some of it in bath water, as a massage oil or as a scent

Mixing equal parts of lavender oil, nutmeg oil and rosemary oil with a carrier oil can be an effective massage oil for aches. Rub it on the upper back and neck area.

Listen to Mellow Sounds or Soft Music - Loud noises can aggravate headaches. Try to listen to softer sounds and relaxing music to calm your senses.

Take Deep Breaths - Breathing lets oxygen to enter and circulate into our air ways, blood, and other organs. Sufficient amount of oxygen is needed in the proper metabolism and other bodily functions.

Improper breathing or shallow breathing decreases the amount of oxygen that enters the body. Deep breathing can help in letting enough oxygen to enter the system.

Insufficient amount of oxygen in the brain can lead to headaches. To relieve headaches, it is a good way to practice deep breathing.

Almonds - Eating almonds can help relieve headaches. It contains some pain-relieving chemicals like salicin, which is one of the ingredients of OTC pain relievers.

Relax Your Shoulder - The way you carry your shoulders can cause some tension on your muscles. If you carry it too high, it may even cause you some headache. Try to drop your shoulders a few times a day to reduce the tension.

Drink Tea - Drinking rosemary, passionflower or lavender tea can help ease headache.

Chamomile or peppermint tea is also effective for relaxation.

Cayenne - You can add some cayenne pepper onto your food. It can also be used topically but with caution. It is an endorphin-stimulant so it can help relieve headaches. It contains capsaicin which is a substance that fights the pain.

To make a cayenne emulsion, just dilute half a teaspoon of powdered cayenne in four oz. of warm water. Mix it with a cotton swab. Put the cotton swab into your nostril to apply the cayenne. This will be a little uncomfortable but it will help relieve your headache.

Stretching Exercises - Stretching can help relieve tension from your neck and shoulders.

Fish Oil Supplements - Some studies show that the intake of fish oil can help improve headache and migraine. The omega-3 fatty acids in fish oil can help reduce inflammations which cause headaches.

Try Feverfew - Feverfew plant contains a substance called parthenolide. It constricts the blood vessels and reduces inflammation thus relieving headaches, especially migraine.

All you need to do is boil a few fresh feverfew flowers in boiling water to make a tea. Let it steep for a few minutes and strain. Drink a cup whenever you have a headache.

Lemon - Lemon juice with tea is a remedy for headache.

You can also pound lemon peel and form it into a paste and put it on your forehead.

Yoga - Yoga is a form of exercise which is known for a lot of stretching, relaxation of the body and calming of the mind. It is a good way to reduce tension which causes headaches.

Get Some Exercise - Moving your body can help relax and loosen up those tight muscles. It might be quite hard to do something when you have a bad headache but believe it or not, it can help reduce your headache.

Try to get some regular exercise if possible. Regular exercise promotes a healthier body.

Appreciate the Outdoors - Try to exercise outside to get some fresh air and a good view of nature. Different scenery can help you to relax and feel better.

Steps to Success Action Plan

Steps to Success has been put together to give you somewhere to start on getting rid of your Headache!

To really have success you may need to use this action plan a few times and trial a few different things to get the result you're after. Test, Measure and Monitor needs to become your motto until you are having headache free days again!

Step 1 - Assess The Severity Of Your Headache.

First of all, you need to assess yourself and measure the intensity of the pain you feel during a headache. You must also carefully identify the type of headache that you are experiencing. The information that I have provided can help you to identify if your headache is a primary or a secondary headache. It can also help you to classify your headache into which type it is.

Step 2- Know The Frequency Of Your Headache.
You must keep a record of your headaches to better keep track of the frequency and duration of your painful headaches. The record can help you to see how many times you experience a headache and on what date or season.
It would be better if you add some notes on each of your entries to help you identify the probable cause of your headache. You can write down the current weather or your whole day activities before the headache occurred.

You can also write down if it is accompanied by an illness.

Step 3 - Visit The Doctor.
After assessing your headache, it is still best to ask a doctor for a proper medication. If he diagnoses your headache as a primary type, you might be well healed by over-the-counter medicines. If he suspects that you have a more serious condition, it would be best to follow his advice.

Step 4 - Resort to Natural Remedies.
If you have been cleared by a doctor from any serious illness, it is good to try natural remedies for headaches. OTC medications may also have side effects and chemical residues.

In trying natural treatments for headaches, you can lessen the chances of other side effects and the intake of toxins.

Step 5 - Change Your Lifestyle.
Your daily activities may be the cause of your headaches. Your daily routine, your habits and your work can be the reason for your headaches.

You can try to get enough rest, avoid stress and keeping a positive outlook in order to lessen the chances of having headaches.
Exercising, proper diet and healthy living can also contribute in keeping your headaches at bay.

Step 6 - Reassess Your Headaches.
After doing all of the previous steps, try to reassess yourself. Write down the improvements, if there is any, after doing or trying out a certain remedy or activity. This way, you can identify which is the best way that can heal your headaches.

Step 7- Seek Medical Attention.
If it happens that after you tried all of the previous steps and there is still no significant improvement, do not hesitate to pay another visit to the doctor. This way you can get a more precise diagnosis for the cause of your headaches and the doctor may prescribe a much better medication or treatment.

Conclusion

Thank you again for downloading this book!

I hope this book was able to help you to identify the causes of your headaches and the possible natural remedies that you can try to heal your headaches. Freeing yourself from headaches can help you to enjoy your life more. It can also help you to be more productive and efficient at work and at your daily activities.

The next step is to put this knowledge to good use and attempt to free yourself from recurring headaches and make the most out of life, you are off to a flying start by reading this book and taking advantage of the Action Plan included.

Finally, if you enjoyed this book, please take the time to share your thoughts and post a review on Amazon. It'd be greatly appreciated!

Thank you and good luck

Other Books you may be interested in...

Below you'll find some of my other books currently available on Amazon. Healthy Body Books now has over 30 books in the series, so jump on line and check them out today!

Manage Your Migraine: The Ultimate Guide to Reducing and Eliminating your Migraines Naturally!

Exercise for Weight loss: 50 Tips to a Happier, Healthier You!

Joint Pain No More: The Most Effective Ways to Eliminate Pain and ease your Aches!

If the links do not work for whatever reason, you can simply search for these amazing titles on the Amazon website.

Free Gift

Thank you again for downloading this Kindle Book Heal Your Headache: The Ultimate Guide to Reducing and Eliminating your Headache Naturally!

I'd like to reward you with this by offering you access to my others books for free by joining my newsletter!

You will be getting up to date information on health, fitness and diet, and also get access to getting other Healthy Body Books for free. By joining my newsletter you will be taking a big step forward in being your Healthiest Body yet!

Just visit **http://www.healthybodybooks.com** and get free instant access to the Healthy Body Books newsletter today!

Lastly once you finish reading this book would please review this book on Amazon. With your feedback I continue to make this book better and better. Thank you

14262161R00024